THE
NETI POT
FOR
BETTER HEALTH

THE
NETI POT
FOR
BETTER HEALTH

WARREN JEFFERSON

Healthy Living Publications
Summertown, Tennessee

Published in the United States by
Healthy Living Publications
P. O. Box 99
Summertown, TN 38483
1-888-260-8458

www.bookpubco.com

Printed in Canada
12 11 10 09 08   9 8 7 6 5

On the cover:
Neti pot available from
The Himalayan Institute,
Hinesdale, PA

The model is
Gretchen Bates

Library of Congress Cataloging-in-Publication Data

Jefferson, Warren, 1943-
  The neti pot for better health / Warren Jefferson.
    p. cm.
  Includes bibliographical references.
  ISBN-13: 978-1-57067-186-9
  ISBN-10: 1-57067-186-9
  1. Nose--Care and hygiene. 2. Nose--Diseases--Alternative treatment. 3. Sinusitis--Alternative treatment. 4. Hay fever--Alternative treatment. 5. Respiratory infections--Alternative treatment. 6. Respiratory allergy--Alternative treatment. 7. Traditional medicine--India. 8. Self-help techniques. I. Title.
  RF354.J44 2005
  616.2'106--dc22   2005026378

The Book Publishing Co. is a member of Green Press Initiative. We have elected to print this title on paper with postconsumer recycled content and processed chlorine free, which saved the following natural resources:

BOOK
PUBLISHING
COMPANY

7 trees
309 lbs of solid waste
2,406 gallons of water
580 lbs of greenhouse gases
5 million BTUs

green
press
INITIATIVE

For more information visit: www.greenpressinitiative.org. Savings calculations thanks to the Environmental Defense Paper Calculator at www.papercalculator.org

CONTENTS

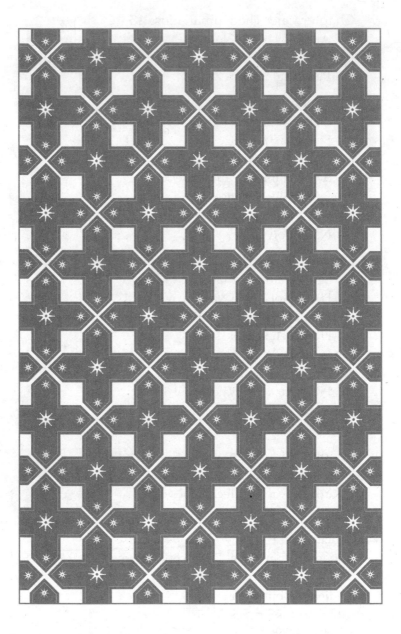

FOREWORD

I have been using the neti pot for a few years now and have become convinced that it is a powerful tool for health. I use my neti pot regularly and have seen a big improvement in my respiratory function.

My mother smoked cigarettes for more than twenty-five years, and I was exposed to secondhand smoke the whole time I was growing up. To make matters, worse as a young man I smoked for 10 years. It won't come as a surprise to know that I have been plagued with respiratory problems (asthma, stuffy nose, and hay fever).

As a result of having a stuffy nose, I was forced to breathe through my mouth during the night and through allergy season. Many health professionals believe that breathing through the mouth can lead to a number of health problems.

I am happy to say that since using the neti pot my condition has improved, and I have been able to breath through my nose most of the time. Hay fever is not the problem it was in years past and if it does begin to develop I use the neti pot and it quickly clears up.

I still struggle with asthma, but I am hopeful that this condition will improve with long-term use of the neti pot, breathing techniques I have learned during my research for this book, and other natural treatments.

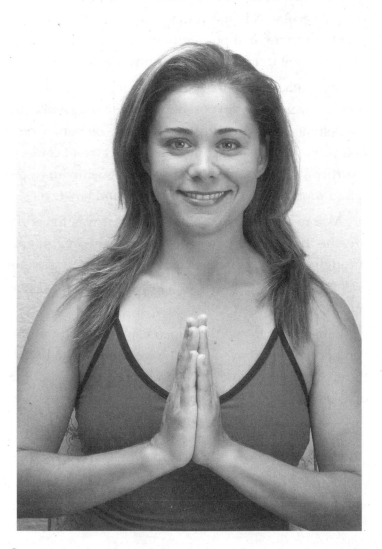

INTRODUCTION

Using the neti pot will help you maintain nasal health and fight off colds and flu. The neti pot used with a saline solution has been shown to be an effective treatment for hay fever, sinusitis, and other nasal conditions.

In the East, Neti, or nasal cleansing, is a common practice that has been in use for thousands of years. Today many people in the West have taken up a modified type of Neti practice called Jala Neti (water neti) using a neti pot. The number of people using the neti pot is growing at a phenomenal rate.

It's not surprising that so many people have adopted the practice of Jala Neti with the neti pot. Chemical air pollution is a growing problem in many parts of the world, and the cases of sinusitis are at an all-time high. People are looking for a way to soothe their troubled noses that doesn't include side effects. Many people believe they have found the help they need using the neti pot.

In *The Neti Pot for Better Health* you will learn:

- detailed methods for using the neti pot to maintain nasal health;
- the symptoms and available treatments for sinusitis;
- the history of saline nasal irrigation in fighting disease and maintaining health;
- the neti pot's long history of use in the East;
- the spiritual aspects of the neti pot and how it is used to enhance meditation;
- where to locate medical resources for treating allergies and other respiratory conditions; and
- how to find neti pot suppliers.

We pay scant attention to our nose unless there are problems, but the nose is an important organ and its proper functioning is essential to health and well-being. The nose is the gateway to the lungs—twelve to sixteen breaths pass through it each minute, twenty-four hours a day. The nose conditions and analyzes each breath. Air is warmed, humidified, and filtered before it ever reaches the lungs.

Our nose is a primary sense organ and gives us important information about our environment. Located here are the smell receptors, which alert us to dangers like fire or other harmful situations. These receptors play a critical role in our ability to taste various flavors in the food we eat. Also in the nose are pheromone receptors, which give us signals about the emotional state of the people around us—are they happy, sad, angry, or receptive?

But the sad fact is our noses are under assault by the very air we breathe. As chemical air pollution increases in many cities throughout the world, we see an epidemic of sinus conditions and asthma developing. Many of us live with a stuffy nose throughout the year and seek relief with the latest decongestant sprays and pills, without much success.

Fortunately there is a simple and economical home remedy available. Medical research and ancient practice have shown saline nasal irrigation (SNI) to be an effective way to maintain nasal health and treat a number of conditions without side effects.

Nasal irrigation is a common practice in many parts of the world. In India nasal irrigation is called Jala Neti (water neti). It is a time-honored technique of personal hygiene that has been used in Ayurveda medicine and Hatha Yoga for thousands of years. Practitioners now use a device called a neti pot to deliver a saline solution to the nasal passages.

The neti pot was introduced to the West approximately thirty years ago and has continued to grow in popularity as yoga has become a common practice for many and as the benefits of SNI have been recognized by Western medicine. With the daily use of the neti pot, a person can maintain nasal health and treat colds, hay fever, and sinusitis, if any of these develop. There is mounting scientific evidence that SNI can have a beneficial effect on the whole respiratory system.

SNI using a neti pot, which I'll refer to simply as "Neti" throughout the book, is a simple procedure that anyone can learn. Thousands of people in North America and western Europe use the neti pot as part of their morning cleansing ritual along with showering and brushing the teeth.

THE
NETI POT
FOR
BETTER HEALTH

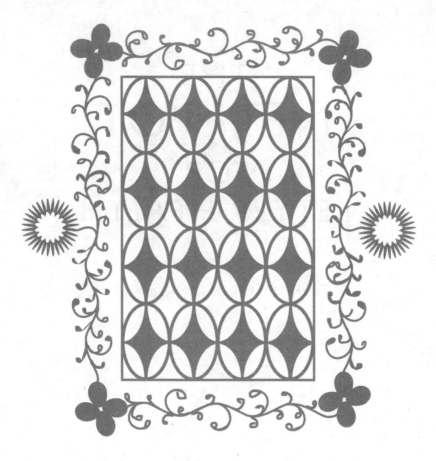

CHAPTER
ONE

THE HUMAN NOSE

ANATOMY
SENSE OF SMELL
PARANASAL SINUSES

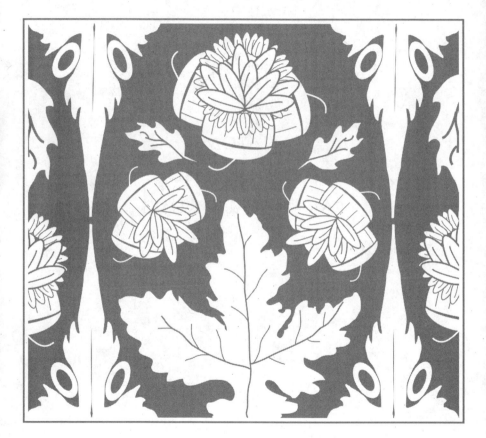

ANATOMY OF THE NOSE

The nose is the main entryway to the respiratory system. With every breath we take, our nose filters, warms, and moistens air entering the lungs (10,000 liters per day). It is the primary organ of smell.

Inside the nose is the nasal cavity, which is divided into two passages by the nasal septum. These two passages open into the nasopharynx, which connects to the throat. Just inside the nose are stiff hairs that trap large airborne particles that might enter. On the surface of the septum is a series of folds, or rounded projections, called turbinates. There are three, one above the other, extending the length of the nasal cavity. They increase the surface area and add turbulence to air passing through the nose, thus moderating its temperature and humidity.

The nasal passages are lined with a blood-rich mucous membrane (mucosa) that secretes mucus. Mucus is the body's first line of defense against disease. It's a clear, wet, slightly sticky substance that contains antiseptic enzymes. It traps small airborne particles and kills harmful microorganisms before they reach the lungs.

In the mucosa also are cilia cells. These specialized cells have a hairlike structure projecting from their surfaces. The cilia move in a coordinated fashion to transport mucus, with its trapped dirt and bacteria, back toward the throat to be swallowed and passed into the stomach for further elimination. Connected to the nasopharynx are the sinus cavities, tear ducts, and eustachian (inner ear) tubes, which all share this mucosa.

As we breathe, air does not flow equally through each nostril. The nose has a periodic cycle in which one side is freely passing air to the lungs while the other side is restricting air. This type of automatic body cycle is technically called an infradian rhythm.

Beneath the mucous membrane is a thick spongy layer called erectile tissue, which contains thousands of microscopic passageways that can fill with blood. There are only three places in the body where this tissue is located: the nose, the genitals, and the breasts.

During this cycle the erectile tissue lining one side of the nose receives increased blood flow, causing the tissue to swell and close off the passageway. At the same time, the other side is losing its supply of blood and is opening and allowing airflow. The cycle then reverses. This natural biological rhythm happens approximately every two hours and is sometimes mistaken for a stuffed up nose.

There is a school of yoga whose focus is the science of breath. They believe that the breath is the connection between the body and the mind, and that if you control the breath you gain control of the mind. They have

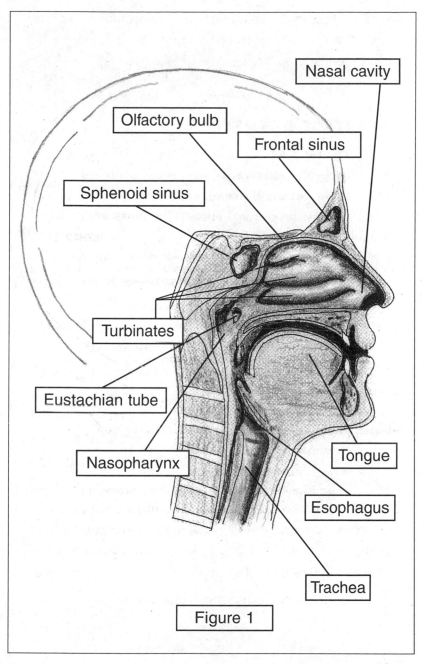

Figure 1

studied this cycle of airflow and consciously control and direct it in an effort to bring about higher self-awareness and spirituality.

THE SENSE OF SMELL

Our sense of smell is not well understood by science and is unappreciated by most of us. But if you lost your sense of smell, your experience of the world would be much poorer. Think of the pleasure of entering a house filled with aromas from dinner cooking, or the wonderful fragrances of a field of wildflowers.

Odor detection by the nose is almost an automatic process. As we breathe, the nose continually samples the air environment for the presence of danger, like smoke, or the presence of food, other people, or animals.

The nose also plays a big part in our sense of taste. How something tastes is in large measure related to how it smells. Do you recall how food tastes bland when you have a cold? Science has determined that we can recognize seven distinct tastes, but the average person can detect ten thousand odors.

We have two chemical senses—smell and taste. The olfactory system, located in the nose, is the sensory system that detects odors. The system is made up of the olfactory epithelium, olfactory bulb, and olfactory nerves.

The olfactory epithelium contains the actual cells

that detect odors, along with supporting cells. It's located along the roof of the nasal cavity, about three inches above and inside the nostrils. It's about one inch wide by three inches long and contains close to 50 million receptor cells. This specialized tissue contains three types of cells: olfactory receptor neurons, cells that protect the neurons and secrete mucus, and basal cells that replace dead neurons.

The sensation of smell occurs when the olfactory receptors are stimulated by contact with gas molecules that pass over them during the process of breathing and sniffing. The chemical property of the molecule is transduced by the olfactory neurons into an electrical signal and sent to the olfactory bulb. From there it is sent directly to the brain, where it is perceived as an odor. The olfactory nerve and the optic nerve are the only nerves that have a direct connection to the brain.

The olfactory epithelium can be damaged by inhaling toxic fumes, by physical injury to the nose, and by the overuse of some nasal sprays. Fortunately, most damage to this tissue is temporary, because this tissue is unique in its ability to regenerate damaged or dead receptor neuron cells, which are replaced every forty days.

Chemicals have specific characteristics, one of which is odor. In order to be detected by the nose, a chemical molecule must be small enough to be volatile and vaporize in the air. Upon reaching the nose, the molecules are dissolved in the mucus and detected by the olfactory neurons. The sinuses in animals with an acute sense of smell are lined with olfactory cells, increasing the surface area available to detect odors. Humans do not have these olfactory cells in the sinuses, which is why our sense of smell is not as acute as certain other animals.

Our sense of smell is a powerful tool of perception and can give us clues about what is in our distant environment. Some flowers emit plumes of odor that can travel on the wind and be detected by honeybees a kilometer away.

In addition to odor receptors, the human nose also contains pheromone receptors. Pheromones are chemicals given off by an organism to communicate with its environment, especially for the purpose of reproduction. Animals and insects communicate and attract each other with pheromones. The queen honeybee communicates with other members of the hive through pheromones. A female silkworm can attract a male silkworm more than two kilometers away with her pheromones.

Humans give off pheromones as well, depending on the kind of emotion they are experiencing. Fear, contentment, and sexual arousal can all be detected by special cells in the nose.

The olfactory nerve terminates in a portion of the brain that is close to an area associated with memory. Research has shown that certain smells can evoke memories rich in vivid detail of events that happened long ago.

Unfortunately, our sense of smell diminishes as we age, and in the elderly it can be reduced by as much as 50 percent. Thick mucus and mucus buildup can hamper the olfactory and pheromone receptors. Avoid prolonged use of over-the-counter nasal decongestant sprays that may damage the cilia. These sprays can become addictive and cause rebound swelling of the nasal passages. Instead, use over-the-counter saltwater nasal mists and sprays.

While traveling via air, carry a spray bottle of saline nasal mist and use it frequently during a long flight. The recycled air in the cabin of airliners is quite dry and could contain a high concentration of cold and flu germs and mold spores. I also recommend using the neti pot after attending a party or large gathering of people.

In order to keep the nose healthy, use the neti pot on a regular basis. Your food will taste better, you will be able to enjoy the pleasant aromas of the day, and you might just pick up the friendly and receptive pheromones from someone you would like to get to know.

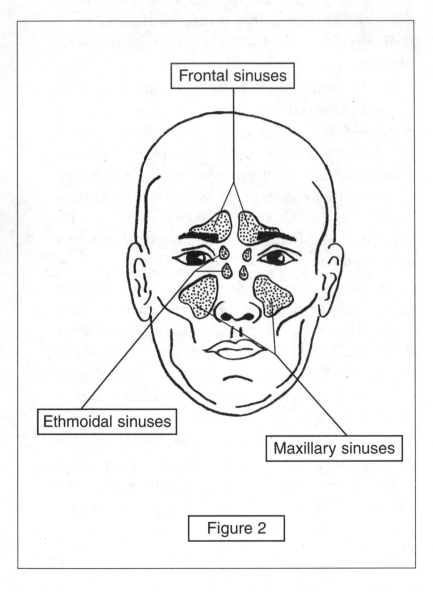

Frontal sinuses

Ethmoidal sinuses

Maxillary sinuses

Figure 2

PARANASAL SINUSES

The paranasal sinuses, commonly referred to as sinuses, are air-filled, mucosal-lined cavities situated in the facial and cranial bones. There are four sets of sinuses lying on each side of the nose. They have a small opening at one end (the ostium) that connects with the nasal passages.

Being air-filled cavities, the sinuses help to decrease the weight of the skull while maintaining its strength and shape. The air spaces of the nose and sinuses add resonance and volume to our voices.

Science does not totally agree on the function of the sinuses. According to some theories, the sinuses help to further trap incoming airborne pollutants that are then moved by the cilia into the nasal cavity through the sinus openings and into the nose and throat for elimination.

The sinus openings are very small and sometimes get blocked by swelling of the mucous membranes brought on by colds or allergies. A blockage can also be caused by abnormal tissue obstruction called polyps. This blockage can lead to sinus inflammation and infection called sinusitis.

There are four different groups of sinuses named for the bones in which they lie:

- frontal: paired and located in the forehead, above the eyebrows

- maxillary: paired and located in the cheek bones, below the eyes

- ethmoid: numerous and somewhat symmetrical, located between the eyes

- sphenoid: paired and located deep in the head at the back of the nose, behind the eyes

Although their function is obscure, problem sinuses can have a profound effect on our health and well-being. Studies have shown that sinus sufferers rate factors such as bodily pain and social functioning as more debilitating with sinusitis than with diseases such as angina, emphysema, chronic bronchitis, and back pain.

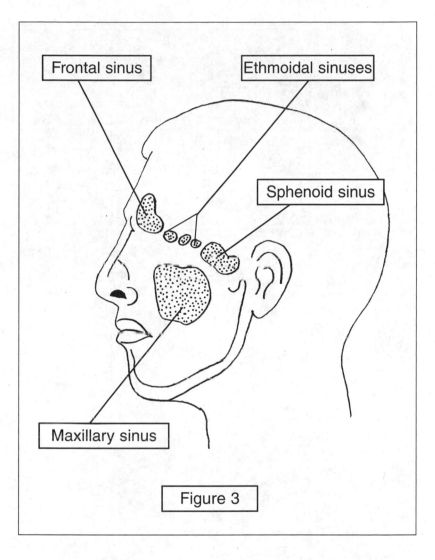

Frontal sinus

Ethmoidal sinuses

Sphenoid sinus

Maxillary sinus

Figure 3

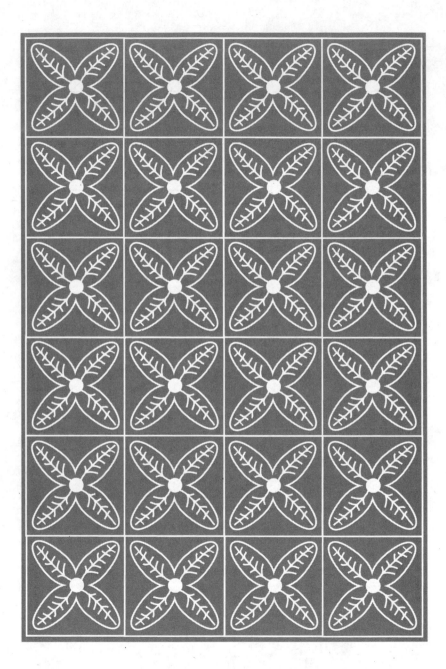

CHAPTER
TWO

NASAL PROBLEMS

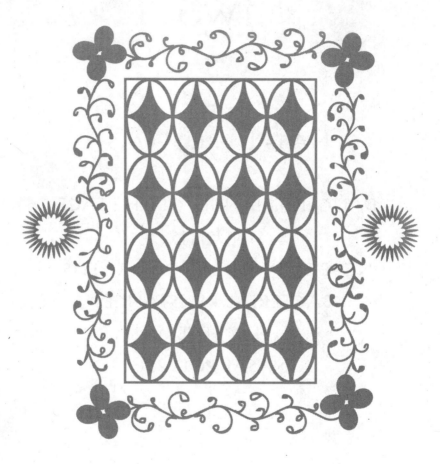

DANGER TRIANGLE OF THE FACE

The nose is one of the few organs of the body that regularly comes in contact with the outside environment; thus the opportunity for invasion by disease agents is always present. Yoga science calls it the "seven paths," because it is the confluence of seven openings of the body: two nostrils, two tear ducts, two eustachian tubes (the inner ear), and the pharynx (upper throat). Hatha Yoga stresses internal cleansing techniques like Neti for increased health maintenance.

The nose is in the center of what Western medicine calls the danger triangle of the face. It's the area from the corners of the mouth to the bridge of the nose, including the nose and maxilla, or upper jaw. Due to the special nature of the blood supply to this area of the body, it is possible for retrograde infections from this area to spread to the brain.

Blood from the danger triangle of the face drains to the rear of the head, where it joins other veins, including veins that drain out of the brain. If an infection occurred here and traveled inward, causing circulation to be blocked, it would cause a life-threatening condition and require surgery. So be very careful when trimming your nose hairs and never pull them out.

SINUSITIS

Sinusitis is an inflammation or swelling of the lining of the sinuses. According to recent estimates, chronic sinusitis affects more than 37 million Americans and results in billions of dollars in health care costs each year.

If the normal drainage of the sinuses is blocked, the cavities can fill with mucus, creating a breeding place for bacteria. Sinus blockage can be caused by the common cold, allergic rhinitis (hay fever), nasal polyps, or mold allergies.

In all cases of sinusitis the goal is to reestablish drainage and clear up infection, if present. Many cases of chronic sinusitis are associated with allergies, so efforts should be focused on the elimination of food or airborne allergens and treatment for the underlying causes of the allergy.

Sinusitis can involve one or more sinuses and can be acute, chronic, or recurrent, and very problematic.

Major symptoms include:

- nasal congestion/blockage
- yellow-green mucus discharge
- swelling around the eyes or cheek
- postnasal drip
- recurring pain near the eyes and front of the head

• partial or complete loss of sense of smell (hyposmia/anosmia)

Minor symptoms include:

• headache

• halitosis (bad breath)

• fatigue

• fever

• cough that may be more severe at night

• ear pain or pressure

Headaches are not a primary symptom of sinus problems, and many migraine headaches are misdiagnosed as sinus headaches. The difference is that a sinus headache is associated with a yellow-green discharge from the nose and the throat, while migraines have a clear discharge, if any.

Many cases of acute sinusitis have their origin in the common cold, which is caused by a virus. Invasion by a virus can inflame the sinuses, because the nose reacts by producing mucus and sending white blood cells to the lining of the nose. The openings of the sinuses can become closed, trapping mucus and bacteria. The trapped bacteria multiply, leading to sinusitis.

Most cases of acute, uncomplicated sinusitis are easily diagnosed and are generally treated with decongestants, painkillers, when needed, and antiallergenic medications, if indicated. The healing process can be accelerated with Neti.

If an infection is present, antibiotics may be needed, but they are not necessary in every case of acute sinusitis. Whenever possible, the body should be given the chance to heal itself without the use of antibiotics. A growing body of research indicates that antibiotics are ineffective in treating acute and chronic sinusitis.

If you must take antibiotics to control your sinusitis, be sure to follow the prescribed course. Do not stop early because you feel better. This could lead to developing antibiotic-resistant bacteria in your system and a more serious infection (see page 38).

Acute sinusitis can also be caused by a fungal infection. People with depressed immune systems can have an allergic reaction to the fungi, causing inflammation of the linings of the nasal passage. There is mounting evidence that allergies may be a major cause of sinusitis, and there seems to be a relationship between having asthma and sinusitis. Seventy-five percent of people with asthma get sinusitis.

Chronic or recurring sinusitis, a condition in which symptoms of an infection persist longer than twelve weeks, needs to be treated differently from acute sinusitis. Standard X-rays can ascertain the presence of acute sinusitis, but to really understand what is going on with problem sinuses, computer tomography (CT scan) is needed. It gives a much better look at the anatomy of the sinuses and the surrounding tissue, and the progression of the disease.

A CT scan can be used along with nasal endoscopy to determine the severity of the condition. A sinus endoscope is a fiber-optic viewing instrument, about the diameter of a straw, with a wide-angle lens at the end. It's inserted into the nose to examine the interior passages.

A simple home test can be performed to determine if your frontal sinuses are blocked. A bright, focused light source (such as a magneto flashlight) can be held against the upper cheek close to the nose. The skin over the sinuses is thin, and if the sinuses are normal, a red dot can be seen on the roof of the mouth (palate), indicating they are air-filled and not obstructed.

The symptoms for acute and chronic sinusitis are similar:

- tender and swollen areas around the affected sinuses
- swollen and red nasal mucous membranes
- runny nose, with possible yellow or green mucus

Pain is generally located around the particular sinus:

- frontal sinusitis: pain in the forehead when touched

- maxillary sinusitis: pain in the cheekbone below the eyes, toothache, and headache in the frontal area

- ethmoid sinusitis: pain between the eyes; headache in the frontal area that can be very intense; swelling of the eyelids and tissue around the eyes; stuffy nose; loss of smell

- sphenoid sinusitis: pain in frontal area, often not localized and felt over several areas.

NOSE BLOWING AND SINUSITIS

Nose blowing may cause sinusitis. A joint study between the University of Virginia and the University of Aarhus in Denmark showed that mucus is propelled into the sinuses during vigorous nose blowing. Coughing or sneezing did not cause nasal mucus to be deposited in the sinuses.

The pressure in the nasal passages while blowing the nose was much higher, 66 mgHg, compared to 5–6 mgHg during sneezing or coughing. That is ten times the amount of pressure, which is capable of propelling one milliliter of nasal mucus into the sinuses. This has serious implications, because this mucus can contain viruses and bacteria, as well as agents that cause inflammation.

So what are we to do when we have a runny nose? Just sniff? Some researchers think that when blowing the nose we should squeeze one nostril closed, which reduces the nasal pressure by half. (Be sure to still blow softly and gently!) Others recommend sniffing mucus to the back of the throat and spitting it out or swallowing it.

Whatever you do, do not squeeze both nostrils closed while you blow. You will not clear the nose properly, and you could cause mucus to be propelled into the sinuses or eustachian tubes, where it could cause an infection.

In a published study, Swedish scientists report they have discovered that humming increases ventilation of the sinuses. They tested a group of ten healthy males, ages thirty-four to thirty-eight, before and after humming, and found that humming sped up the exchange of air between the sinuses and nasal cavity. This may be one of the benefits of chanting Om.

SWOLLEN INFERIOR TURBINATE

As mentioned earlier, there are three turbinates that line each side of the nasal septum and run parallel to the nasal passage. They are referred to as the superior, middle, and inferior turbinates. Because of its position, the inferior turbinate could cause a nasal blockage if it becomes swollen.

An enlarged or swollen inferior turbinate could be caused by allergies, irritant exposure, sinus inflammation, or a deformed nasal septum that causes the bone to enlarge. If the enlargement is related to allergies, treating the allergies and doing Neti will usually solve the problem. If treatment does not reduce the enlargement, reduction surgery may be necessary.

Modern procedures using endoscopic surgery can reduce the size of the underlying bone structure and selectively remove tissue, if necessary, with few complications. A persistently swollen inferior turbinate can be treated with a freezing technique (cryotherapy) or heated with a radio frequency current (cautery or radiofrequency surgery).

BACTERIAL RESISTANCE

The bacteria that cause most upper respiratory infections (Streptococcus pneumoniae, Haemophilus influenzae, and Moraxella catarrhalis) have become resistant to antibiotics due to their misuse and overuse in the treatment of sinusitis. This particular type of bacterial resistance has increased 40–50 percent in the last twenty years. The National Institute of Allergy and Infectious Diseases (NIAID) recently declared:

> Drug-resistant infectious agents—those that are not killed or inhibited by antimicrobial

compounds—are an increasingly important public health concern. Tuberculosis, gonorrhea, malaria, and childhood ear infections are just a few of the diseases that have become more difficult to treat due to the emergence of drug-resistant pathogens. Antimicrobial resistance is becoming a factor in virtually all hospital-acquired infections. Many physicians are concerned that several bacterial infections soon may be untreatable (2000).

The report goes on to say that the costs for treating antibiotic-resistant infections in the United States may be as high as $30 billion.

Streptococcus pneumoniae, the disease microbe that causes thousands of cases of meningitis and pneumonia and millions of cases of ear infections (and sinusitis) in the United States each year, is developing resistance to penicillin, the drug of choice by most doctors. Unfortunately, many of these penicillin-resistant strains are also resistant to other antibiotics.

Guidelines to address this problem have been issued by the Centers for Disease Control and Prevention (CDC). They were developed to assist health professionals to more accurately diagnose acute bacterial rhinosinusitis (ABRS) and to use the most effective treatment. The guidelines analyze and rank seventeen antibiotics used to treat sinusitis by how effective they are in fighting the bacteria that most often cause this condition.

Doing Neti on a regular basis has been shown to aid nasal health. Practitioners claim that many problems with the upper respiratory system can be prevented or improved by doing Neti daily.

HAY FEVER

Allergic rhinitis, called hay fever or allergies when it occurs seasonally, is a condition suffered by close to 40 million Americans. It is especially troublesome in the spring and summer months. Seasonal allergic rhinitis is commonly caused by plant pollen from ragweed, grass, trees, and mold spores. Ragweed pollen accounts for more than 75 percent of the cases of seasonal allergic rhinitis. There is also a condition called perennial allergic rhinitis in which symptoms occur throughout the year. It is caused by an allergen that is present continuously in the environment.

Allergic rhinitis is a condition in which the body's oversensitized immune system reacts to dust, dander, and pollen and creates a misdirected immune response. This produces a release of histamines, a body chemical, into the bloodstream, causing itchy eyes, swollen nasal tissue, hives, rashes, increased mucus production, and other symptoms. These symptoms can be mild to severe, depending on the person affected, but do not endanger general health.

Neti has been shown to help with this condition. The International Consensus Report on the Diagnosis and Management of Rhinitis recommends nasal irrigation as a treatment for allergic rhinitis. Rhinitis is often associated with asthma and other allergy disorders. Controlling the symptoms of hay fever can aid in the treatment of asthma.

NASAL POLYPS

Nasal polyps are small growths on the mucous membrane and are formed from an overproduction of mucus. They look like pearly gray lumps and typically lie deep in the nasal passage. They are generally harmless, unless they protrude into the sinus openings and cause blockage and infection or restrict airflow in the nasal passage and make breathing difficult.

If you notice your breathing becoming increasingly congested over time, you may have nasal polyps. The traditional treatment is to have them surgically removed. But depending on the cause, Neti, along with specific herbs, could help by improving circulation and restoring the mucous membrane to health.

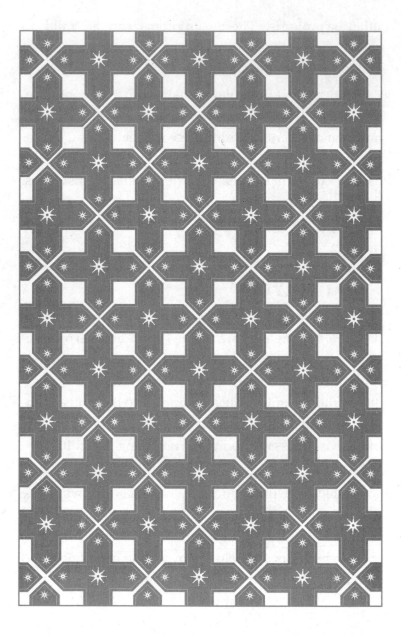

CHAPTER
THREE

USING THE
NETI POT

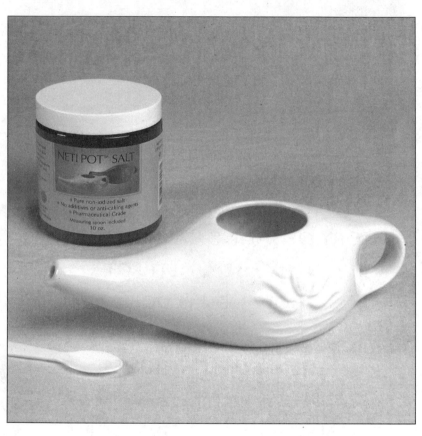

Figure 4

SALT—NATURE'S ANTISEPTIC

The use of a neti pot requires mixing up a saline solution (salt and water) that will be poured through the nasal passages. Salt is an antiseptic and has been used for thousands of years to fight infection. An ancient Egyptian papyrus thought to be from Imhotep, a famous builder and doctor (300 BCE), describes the treatment of a chest wound with salt. It was believed that salt would dry out the wound and disinfect it. Later, many salt recipes in the form of suppositories, liquids, and ointments were used to treat a wide variety of diseases.

The ancient Greek physician Hippocrates (460 BCE) used salt preparations, including saltwater steam inhalations, to treat diseases. A mixture of salt and vinegar was recommended to clean acute ulcers, and ocean-bath therapy was used to cure skin diseases.

In ancient Rome, the medical book *De Materia Medica*, by the military doctor Dioscorides of the first century CE, recommends salty vinegar be used to treat dog bites and the bites of poisonous animals, and as a laxative. Roman doctors used salt preparations to treat a variety of ailments and maladies. *De Materia Medica* was the precursor to all modern pharmacopeias and remained in use until 1600.

Blood, sweat, and tears contain salt, and both the skin and the eyes are protected from infectious germs by the antibacterial properties of salt. In the proper strength, it kills or prevents the growth and reproduction of most microorganisms it comes in contact with, including bacteria, fungi, protozoa, and viruses. We all know to gargle with warm salt water for a sore throat.

Therapeutic salt solutions can vary in concentration, which is referred to as tonicity or salinity. There are two medically useful salt solutions: the isotonic chloride solution and the hypertonic chloride solution.

An isotonic solution has the same salt salinity as the blood plasma of vertebrates, approximately 0.9 percent, and is called normal saline. There are nine grams of salt in one liter of water. Hypertonic saline solutions include 1.8 percent, 3 percent, 5 percent, 7.5 percent, and 10 percent sodium chloride concentrations.

Normal saline can be injected intravenously, subcutaneously, or intramuscularly. It is used to save the lives of accident victims, as it can temporarily replace lost blood. It can also be used to replace gastric juices in cases of digestive disease, and is used as an irrigation fluid during many surgeries. This solution is about four times less salty than seawater.

Both the isotonic and hypertonic chloride solutions are used for Neti. For daily use, an isotonic solution is best; but for treating allergic rhinitis or hay fever, a hypertonic solution can sometimes be helpful in reducing the swelling of nasal membranes associated with this condition.

There is evidence that a hypertonic solution, which has a higher concentration of salt, can help shrink swollen membranes by a process of osmosis, allowing freer breathing and drainage of the sinuses. A hypertonic solution should be buffered before use so its pH matches the body's to prevent stinging in the nasal passages. There are hypertonic salt-buffer mixtures available commercially from many outlets.

HISTORY OF SALINE NASAL IRRIGATION

European physicians in the nineteenth century encouraged their patients to use saline nasal irrigation (SNI) for health maintenance and routine cleansing. In North America it has been a folk remedy to treat colds and flu for more than a hundred years. There is growing scientific evidence that nasal irrigation is effective in treating many conditions affecting the nose, with no side effects.

In modern times, saline nasal irrigation has become more widely accepted as a home remedy to relieve conditions such as allergies, colds, mild sinus infections, and hay fever. Science has studied SNI for the treatment of a number of other nasal conditions including occupational irritants, the common cold, post-treatment for nasal surgery, and cystic fibrosis. Most of these conditions see improvement with SNI. Preliminary research indicates that SNI could also be an effective treatment for allergic rhinitis and chronic sinusitis.

Science does not know exactly how SNI works, but theories include the following:

- mechanical clearing of mucus
- improved functioning of cilia
- decreased swelling of the mucous membrane
- decreased mucus production
- removal of irritants that could cause inflammation

There are advantages to using SNI instead of over-the-counter and prescribed drugs to treat nasal problems:

- saline solution has a soothing effect on the nasal membranes
- antibiotics are not being used, thus friendly flora are not destroyed
- SNI is less expensive
- SNI has no side effects, such as drowsiness or upset stomach
- SNI is well tolerated, and with the right balance of salt and water, there is no stinging

Various forms of nasal irrigation being used in clinical trials include:

- saline lavage using a large capacity syringe
- humidified warm air lavage, known as hyper thermia
- nebulized aerosol therapy using saline solution

Other uses have been suggested for SNI, but none have been thoroughly studied in humans and there is little scientific evidence as to their effectiveness. SNI has not been shown to be an effective treatment for asthma, chronic bronchitis, or nasal polyps. Some of these conditions are potentially life-threatening and should be treated by a qualified medical professional.

WHY USE A NETI POT?

It may seem strange and unnatural to run salt water through your nose, but consider this. There are 32 million cases of sinusitis reported to the U.S. Centers for Disease Control (CDC) annually. Sinusitis is one of the most common health care complaints in the United States and costs the economy $3.5 billion annually. During the summer months, most large cities in the United States do not meet the Environmental Protection Agency standards for air quality. It seems that over the years, as the level of air pollution has gone up, so have the reported cases of sinusitis.

SNI can be done effectively using a small pot called a neti pot. A mild saline solution is mixed, put in the neti pot, and poured through the nasal passages—first one side, then the other. (For a more complete description, see the section that follows.)

The flow of warm, slightly salty water removes old mucus, and with it trapped dirt and germs. Thus the nose is thoroughly cleansed and refreshed, and the breath is free-flowing. Practitioners claim it also has a beneficial effect on the eyes, ears, throat, lungs, and mind.

SNI with a neti pot is a simple, low-cost, and effective way to keep the nose and sinuses healthy. It takes less than ten minutes from start to finish, but it could be the single most important daily health maintenance program a person can do.

HOW NETI IS DONE

A neti pot is a small container, either metal, ceramic, or plastic, with a tapered spout and an end about the size of an average person's nostril. (See figure 4, page 44.) Neti pots come in various sizes and capacities. The one I use holds about eight ounces or one-quarter liter and is ceramic. It looks like a small Aladdin's lamp.

The neti pot is filled with warm water that is mixed with a small amount of salt. The spout is inserted into a nostril and the head is positioned so that the water, under the force of gravity, flows into one nostril and out the other. In yoga science this type of neti is called Jala Neti Stage I.

The salt to water proportion is important. Use one-quarter teaspoon of salt to eight ounces or one-quarter liter of water. This is close to a normal saline solution and matches the body's concentration of salt. Make sure that the salt is totally dissolved. Use only non-iodized salt, sea salt, halite (rock salt), or kosher salt for your solution. Table salt is not suitable because it contains iodide and other chemicals to keep it free-flowing.

At least four ounces or one-eighth liter of solution should be run through each nostril, although some people like more. (I mix sixteen ounces at a time and run a full pot through each nostril.) The water should be close to body temperature, 98 degrees Fahrenheit, and slightly less salty than seawater. Check the water temperature on your wrist as though you were testing a baby bottle, and taste it for saltiness. It should taste like your tears. Use filtered water when possible, but this is not essential unless your tap water is especially poor quality. With this concentration of salt water close to body temperature, you will hardly notice the solution passing through your nose.

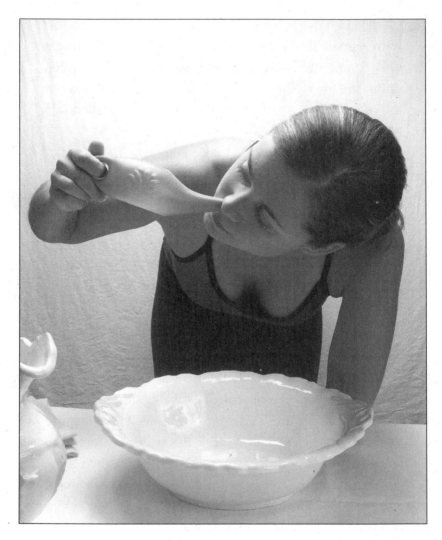

Figure 5

Neti can be done over the bathroom sink, in the shower, over a large catch basin, or outdoors. Assuming you are doing it over the bathroom sink, have a supply of paper towels or tissues handy. Fill the neti pot with the proper mixture of saline solution. Face the sink and bend down at the waist. It doesn't matter which nostril you start with, but you will probably favor one side as you develop your practice.

Turn your head slightly and insert the spout of the neti pot into the upper nostril. Ensure that you have a tight fit. Continue to turn your head until the opposite nostril is pointing down. Angle the nose down as well, so that the lower nostril is slightly lower than your chin. Tilt the back of the pot up slightly while you breathe through your mouth. (See figure 5, facing page.)

In a few seconds, water should begin to flow out of the lower nostril. Continue until half the solution is used. The total time will vary, depending on the condition of your nasal passages. An unobstructed flow of eight ounces through one nostril should take twenty to twenty-five seconds.

Remove the pot, breathe in through your mouth, and blow the air gently out through your nostrils several times to clear water and mucus. Repeat the procedure with the remaining solution for the other nostril. Perform the drying technique (see page 56). If you did not get a good flow through your nasal passages, repeat the process.

There are a number of other devices that can be used to deliver saline solution besides the neti pot:

- squeeze bottle
- large capacity syringe with a special nasal tip (see figure 6 below)
- bulb syringe
- Waterpik® with a special nasal tip
- nasal irrigation system that delivers saline solution with an electrical pump
- the old fashioned way, a cupped hand

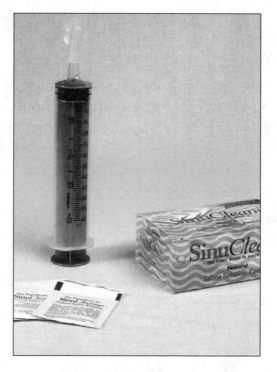

Figure 6

For children, the Waterpik® with a special tip or the pump system might be the only way to effectively deliver saline solution to their small nasal passages. For most adults, the neti pot will work well. It's simple, low-tech, and uses gravity.

Neti is generally done one or two times a day, but it can be done more frequently if needed. The first time should be in the morning, to clear out residue accumulated during the night. Before bed is also a good time, to ensure free breathing during sleep.

HOW THE WATER FLOWS

When doing Neti, the saline solution flows in the first nostril, into the first nasal passage, around the septum, into the middle nasal cavity (nasopharynx), into the other nasal passage, and out the opposite nostril. It should not flow back into the throat during this type of Neti, which is referred to as Stage I Jala Neti in yoga tradition. Stage II Jala Neti is a technique in which water flows in through the nostrils and out the mouth. (See page 68 for a brief explanation.)

As the saline solution flows through the nasal passages, it draws out and dilutes mucus with trapped impurities and flushes it out through the nostrils. The water flow also creates a low-pressure zone (venturi effect) across the sinuses, which helps draw out deeper dirt and mucus and helps keep the sinuses clear. It has a similar effect on the tear ducts and eustachian tubes. After doing Neti for a while, people speak of having sharper vision, brighter eyes, and improved hearing.

DRYING TECHNIQUES

At the end of the Neti process it is important to thoroughly dry the nose. Make sure you have a paper towel or supply of tissues handy. Turn away from the sink, lean forward, and bend at the hips until the top of the head is pointed toward the floor. (See figure 7 below.) Hold this position for about ten seconds. Hold a paper towel or some tissues over your nose to catch the solution that will drip out. This movement will allow any solution farther in the nasopharynx to drain out.

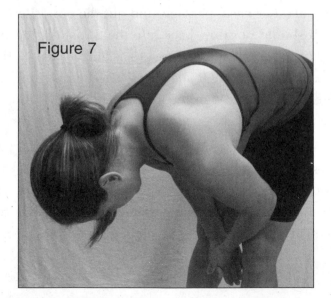

Figure 7

Return to the upright position and lean over the sink. Close one nostril with the middle and ring fingers as shown in figure 8 below, breathe in through the mouth, and blow out gently through the open nostril ten times. Close the other nostril and again blow out gently ten times. (See page 36 for cautions about blowing the nose.)

This should remove any remaining water and loosened mucus from the nasal passages. Do not use forceful exhales through your nose. You do not want to blow moisture or mucus into your sinuses.

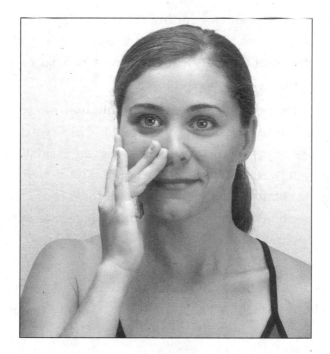

Figure 8

PROBLEMS WITH WATER FLOW

The first few times you do Neti you may not get any water flow through the nostrils or you may get just a trickle. A number of factors could cause this:

- the spout may be pushed against the nasal passage blocking the water flow
- the pot may not be tilted enough
- the angle of the head may be incorrect
- there could be nasal blockage from swollen nasal membranes or thick mucus

Even if you are not getting the proper flow through the nostrils, just having the saline solution in contact with the nasal passage will produce beneficial results. Try the following procedure.

Fill the neti pot with saline solution at the correct temperature. Insert the tip of the neti pot in a nostril and fill one side of your nose with the solution. Hold it there for about twenty seconds while breathing through your mouth. Remove the neti pot and blow out gently through that nostril while holding the other nostril closed with the middle and ring fingers.

Fill the other nostril and hold for about twenty seconds. Breathe through the mouth. Remove the neti pot and blow out gently again, holding the opposite nostril closed with the middle and ring fingers.

Repeat this procedure, first on one side and then the other, three or four times. Be patient and don't get discouraged. If you do this every day for about a week you should get a reasonable amount of flow through your nose. You could also try the nasal syringe shown in fig. 6. I had trouble getting flow through my nose at first and the syringe helped.

If after trying the methods outlined above you still do not get any flow, the blockage may be due to an actual physical condition like polyps (abnormal tissue growths), a deviated septum, or an enlarged turbinate (see page 37). You should consider having a medical professional check you out.

NATURAL ADDITIVES FOR THE NETI POT

In Ayurveda medicine, herbs and oils are sometimes added to the saline solution to soothe and treat conditions of the nasal passages as well as other conditions of the body and mind. The membranes in the nose can absorb the healing aspects of an herb or oil, providing treatment both locally and systemically.

There are herbal extracts and tinctures that have been shown to help cleanse, decongest, and invigorate the nasal passages. They can be added to the saline solution and are available from a number of retailers, including those listed on page 75.

In folk medicine there is also some use of herbal tea as the fluid used to irrigate and treat sinus problems. In his book *Back to Eden*, Jethro Kloss recommends cold applications or alternate cold and hot applications over the sinus, along with a tea of bayberry bark to be inhaled into each nostril for sinus troubles. Kloss states that this will cleanse and heal at the same time.

According to Max Skousen, author of the *Aloe Vera Handbook*, aloe vera juice is helpful for mild sinus problems and a stuffy nose. The method is to fill an empty squeeze-bottle nasal inhaler halfway with stabilized aloe vera juice. Spray the juice into your nose, just as you would a regular antihistamine medicine. Unlike antihistamines, it will not dry out the nose or cause rebound blockage, and it is mild enough to be used as often as needed.

THE BENEFITS OF NETI

Not all the benefits listed below have been con-firmed by scientific research; some are strictly anecdotal. Only by giving Neti a try will you be able to tell whether it will give you relief from your condition. Using a neti pot:

- removes dirt, germs, and pollen from the nose;

- relieves the symptoms of hay fever, such as runny nose and itchy eyes;

- reduces swollen mucous membranes in the nose, allowing free nasal breathing rather than mouth breathing; this in turn adds to the general health of the whole respiratory system and aids in the treatment of asthma and other respiratory diseases;

- helps the sinuses drain and function properly due to a reduction in swelling of the mucous membranes;

- helps create the proper conditions in the nasal passages so the nose can do its job of filtering and conditioning air entering the lungs;

- improves the sense of smell, which can heighten the sense of taste and lead to a healthy appetite;

- can be helpful in treating certain ear infections, reducing the need for antibiotics;

- cools and soothes the brain and gives relief from headaches, depression, and general mental tension;

- has a positive effect on the pineal and pituitary glands, which helps to maintain hormonal and emotional balance.

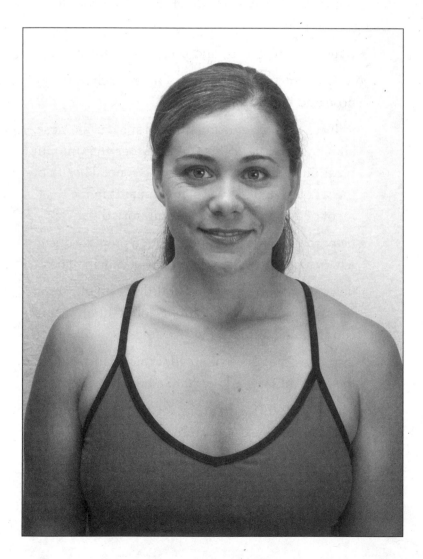

CHAPTER FOUR

4

YOGA AND THE NETI POT

SPIRITUAL ASPECTS OF NETI

YOGA CLEANSING TECHNIQUES

JALA NETI STAGE II

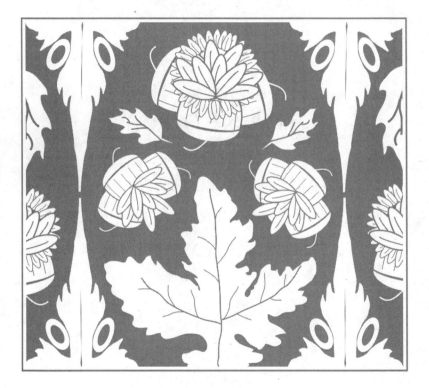

SPIRITUAL ASPECTS OF NETI

In Hatha Yoga the term Neti is used to describe an ancient technique that is somewhat different from the Neti practice we have been discussing. This traditional Neti is one of the six cleansing techniques, or kriyas, that have been practiced in India for thousands of years. It's done with plain water, salt water, or with a special knotted cord. The use of a neti pot is a modern adaptation of this ancient cleansing practice and has been adopted by many modern schools of yoga.

Practitioners believe Neti can help bring about proper breathing, which leads to balance in the body and mind. Yogis use it as part of their personal cleansing ritual, but they also use it to help them attain higher states of meditation leading to enlightenment, transcendence, and some say immortality. It is referenced in ancient yogic texts such as Gheranda Samhita and Hatha Yoga Pradipika.

YOGA CLEANSING TECHNIQUES
From Hatha Yoga Pradipika:

> 20.) By removing the impurities, the air can be restrained, according to one's wish [I interpret this to mean if impurities in the body are removed, one would have more control over the breath] and the appetite is increased, the divine sound is awakened, and the body becomes healthy.

21.) If there be excess of fat or phlegm in the body, the six kinds of kriyas (duties) should be performed first. But others, not suffering from the excess of these, should not perform them.

22.) The six kinds of duties are: Dhauti [stomach cleansing with a cloth], Basti [colonic irrigation], Neti [nasal cleansing with water or a cord], Trataka [cleansing and strengthening the eyes], Nauli [strengthening the rectus-abdominii], and Kapalabhati [respiratory cleansing through forceful breathing]. These are called the six actions.

23.) These six kinds of actions, which cleanse the body, should be kept secret. They produce extraordinary attributes and are performed with earnestness by the best Yogis.

From Hatha Yoga Pradipika describing Neti:

29.) A cord made of threads and about six inches long should be passed through the passage of the nose and the end taken out in the mouth. This is called by adepts the Neti Karma.

30.) The Neti is the cleaner of the brain and giver of divine sight. It soon destroys all the diseases of the cervical and scapular regions.

Practitioners of Neti believe that it helps free the breath and has a positive effect on the mind. In yoga science the energy of the body, called prana, is thought to sustain life. Prana flows throughout the body and through seven centers or chakras. These chakras lie in the center of the body from the groin to the top of the head.

The Ajna Chakra is the sixth chakra. It is situated between the eyebrows, right below the crown of the head. It is thought to control awakening and spiritual vision. This is the same general area where the two sides of the nasal passages join the nasopharynx.

It is believed that the Ajna Chakra is the place where two branches of prana, Ha and Tha, come together. The pituitary gland lies in this region and is thought to be stimulated by Neti. This is the area where the mythical "third eye" lies. According to yoga teaching, when the Ajna Chakra is in balance, mental insight, clairvoyance, self-control, intuition, and extrasensory perception are all possible. It is believed that Neti can help balance the Ajna Chakra.

If you want to explore this area of Neti further, I recommend reading *Science of Breath* by Swami Rama, and *Neti: Healing Secrets of Yoga and Ayurveda* by David Frawley. These books provide good introductions to the subject.

JALA NETI STAGE II

Jala Neti Stage II is a yoga technique in which the flow of water is directed into the nostril and out the mouth. Reportedly it helps clean the inner sinuses and relieves postnasal drip.

Most yoga teachers recommend that Jala Neti Stage II should not be tried until Stage I is mastered. Once you are comfortable doing Stage I you may want to try Stage II. The technique is not difficult, but you have to breathe through your mouth while water is going down the back of your throat and out your mouth. You have to control the gag reflex and maintain an open throat during the process.

The angle of the head is critical in order for the solution to flow through properly. The position is about the same as with Stage I, except the nose is positioned at the same angle as the chin or a little higher. Hold the proper angle, and in a few seconds the water will begin to flow out of your mouth as well as your nose. Not only do the nasal passages get bathed with the soothing saline solution, the inner sinuses and upper throat do as well.

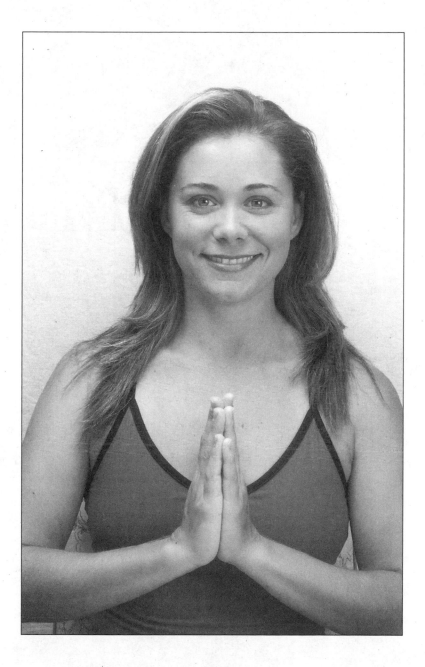

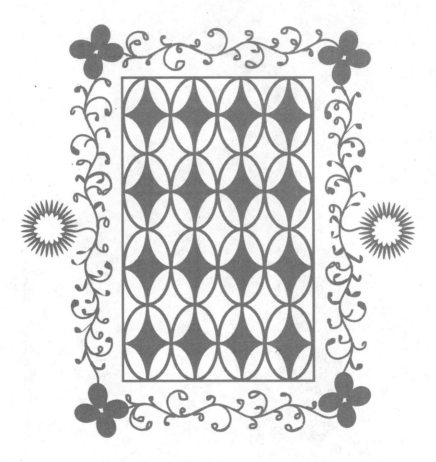

CONCLUSION

The human nose is the gateway to the lungs, and its proper functioning is important to our health and well-being. The nose conditions and analyzes every breath we take, warming, humidifying, and filtering the air before it ever reaches the lungs.

But our noses are under assault by the very air we breathe. Chemical air pollution is increasing worldwide and is causing an epidemic of sinus problems and asthma. Modern research and ancient practice has shown saline nasal irrigation to be an effective treatment for a number of nasal conditions and an excellent way to maintain nasal health.

Saline nasal irrigation is a time-honored practice in many parts of the world. Using the neti pot has become very popular in the West, and many alternative health professionals are recommending it to their sinus patients.

With this book I have attempted to compile the latest knowledge about how to keep the nose healthy and functioning properly using the technique of saline nasal irrigation with the neti pot. I hope you find it helpful. Here's wishing you free-flowing breath.

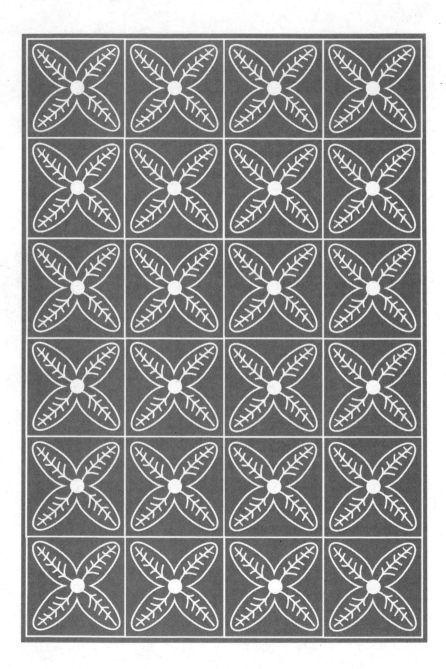

APPENDIX

Functional Endoscopic Sinus Surgery

When chronic sinusitis does not respond to home remedies like Neti, and antibiotics cannot relieve the infection, surgery is required to facilitate drainage and remove pustules and infected mucous membranes. Today, because of advanced technology, most sinus operations are done completely inside the nose.

The operation is called Functional Endoscopic Sinus Surgery (FESS). The procedure involves inserting a small flexible tube containing a miniature camera, a fiber-optic light source, and a miniature surgical instrument into the nasal passage.

FESS is used effectively to remove polyps and other abnormal tissue obstructions in the nose and sinuses. The natural openings of the sinuses can be enlarged where they connect at the nasal passage, while the integrity of the sinus surfaces is maintained.

The benefits of FESS are restored ventilation and natural drainage of the sinus. It can be done with local anesthetic without external incisions, and the procedure can usually be performed as outpatient surgery. Prior to the development of this technique, sinus surgery was performed through external incisions or incisions under the upper lip. The old surgery was more intrusive and destructive to the sinuses and nasal linings; it often required removing the sinuses and creating non-physiological drainage.

FESS usually takes one to two hours and may in some cases require an overnight stay. Nasal packing and plastic implants may be required, which will be removed in about a week during the post-op examination. Pain after the operation is usually not very severe. Complications are rare, but may include one or more of the following: bleeding, fever, infection, or pain, and the operation may not lead to normal functioning of the sinuses. Other complications as a result of the location of the sinuses could include eye problems, diminished sense of smell, and central nervous system problems, but these are very rare and can be dealt with if treated early.

NETI POT, SALT & NASAL WASH SOURCES

Health and Yoga
http://www.healthandyoga.com

Herbal Remedies
http://herbal-remedies-usa.stores.yahoo.net

Himalayan Institute
http://www.netipot.org

Into The Scented Garden
http://www.intothescentedgarden.com

Peaceful Company
http://www.peacefulcompany.com

Yoga Essentials
http://www.yogaessentials.com

MEDICAL RESOURCES

American Academy of Allergy, Asthma, and
Immunology
555 East Wells Street, Suite 1100
Milwaukee, WI 53202
800-822-2762
http://www.aaaai.org

American Academy of Otolaryngology—Head and
Neck Surgery
One Prince Street
Alexandria, VA 22314-3357
703-836-4444
http://www.entnet.org

Asthma and Allergy Foundation of America
1233 20th Street NW, Suite 402
Washington, DC 20036
202-466-7643
http://www.aafa.org

Joint Council of Allergy, Asthma, and Immunology
50 North Brockway, Suite 3-3
Palatine, IL 60067
847-934-1918
http://www.jcaai.org

National Institute of Allergy and Infectious Diseases
National Institutes of Health
Office of Communications and Public Liaison
6610 Rockledge Drive, MSC 6612
Bethesda, MD 20892
301-496-5717
http://www.niaid.nih.gov

National Library of Medicine
MedlinePlus
8600 Rockville Pike
Bethesda, MD 20894
888-346-3656
http://medlineplus.gov

OTHER USEFUL SOURCES

Grossan Hydro Pulse Nasal/Sinus Irrigation System (retail price $89.00). The manufacturer claims that Pulsatile Sinus Irrigation uses a gentle, pulsating stream of saline solution to moisturize the nasal passages, remove foreign matter, crusts, and other undesirable materials, and massage the cilia of the mucous membrane back to health.

http://www.alerg.com

American Academy of Otolaryngology—Head and Neck Surgery. An excellent site for information on all aspects of the nose and sinuses, with 3-D virtual reality illustrations of the nasal passages, sinuses, and FESS surgery techniques.

http://www.entnet.org/healthinfo/sinus/ sinus_home.cfm

For in-depth noncommercial information on Neti, go to: www.jalanetipot.com

REFERENCES

Balch, J., and P. Balch. 1997. *Prescription for Nutritional Healing*. Garden City Park, NY: Avery Publishing Group.

Cayman, C. 1994. *The American Medical Association Family Medical Guide*. New York: Random House.

Frawley, D. 2005. *Neti: Healing Secrets of Yoga and Ayurveda*. Twin Lakes, WI: Lotus Press.

Gheranda. 1996. *Gheranda Samhita*. New Delhi, India: Munshiram Manoharlal Publishers.

Gray, H. 1977. *Gray's Anatomy*. New York: Bounty Books.

Guinness, A., ed. 1993. *Family Guide to Natural Medicine*. Pleasantville, NY: The Readers Digest Association, Inc.

Jefferson, W. 2003. *Colloidal Silver Today*. Summertown, TN: Healthy Living Publications.

Kloss, J. 1939. *Back to Eden*. Loma Linda, CA: Back to Eden Book Publishing Co.

Massachusetts Eye and Ear Infirmary. The Sinuses. http://www.meei.harvard.edu/shared/oto/rhino.php (accessed August 18, 2005).

Merck Manual of Medical Information—Second Home Edition, Online Version. http://www.merck.com/mmhe/index.html (accessed August 18, 2005).

Murray, M., and J. Pizzorno. 1998. *Encyclopedia of Natural Medicine*. Roseville, CA: Prima Health.

National Institute of Allergyand Infectious Diseases. 2000. *Antimicrobial Resistance Fact Sheet*. Bethesda, MD:National Institute of Allergy and Infectious Diseases.

————. 2004. Antimicrobial Resistance. http://www.niaid.nih.gov/publications/antimic.htm (accessed August 18, 2005).

————. 2005. Sinusitis. http://www.niaid.nih.gov/factsheets/sinusitis.htm (accessed August 18, 2005).

Natural Standard and Faculty of Harvard Medical School. 1994. International consensus report on the diagnosis and management of rhinitis: Nasal irrigation. *Allergy* 49:1–34. http://www.naturalstandard.com (accessed August 18, 2005).

Rama, Swami, R. Ballentine, and A. Hymes. 1998. *Science of Breath*. Honesdale, PA: Himalayan Institute Press.

Saraswati, Swami Bhavchaitanya. Neti Introduction, Neti Benefits, Neti In-Depth. http://www.bytheplanet.com/Products/Yoga/neti/Netipot.htm (accessed August 18, 2005).

Shoseyov, D., H. Bibi, P. Shai, N. Shoseyov, G. Shazberg, and H Hurvitz. 1998. Treatment with hypertonic saline versus normal saline nasal wash of pediatric chronic sinusitis. *Journal of Allergy and Clinical Immunology* 101(5):602-5.

Skousen, M. B. 1992. *Aloe Vera Handbook*. Summertown, TN: Healthy Living Publications.

Stamatos, J. M. 2005. *Pain Free*. McKinney, TX: The Magni Company.

Svatmarama. 2002. *Hatha Yoga Pradipika*. Woodstock, NY: YogaVidya.com.

West Virginia University. Diseases of the Nose and Sinuses. http://www.hsc.wvu.edu/som/otolaryngology/ diseases/nose.htm (accessed August 18, 2005).

Wormer, E. J. 1999. A Taste for Salt in the History of Medicine.http://www.tribunes.com/tribune/sel/ worm.htm (accessed August 18, 2005).

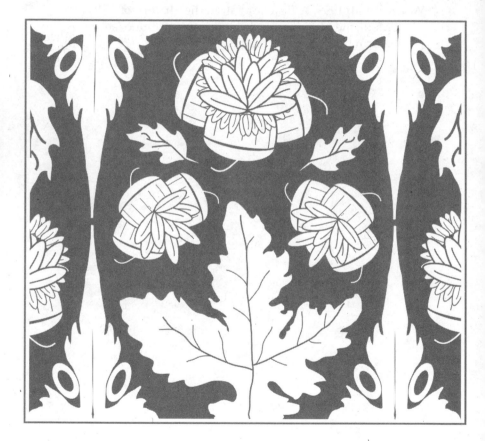

INDEX

A

acute bacterial rhinosinusitis (ABRS), 39
additives, to the neti pot, 60
air pollution
    damage to olfactory system, 21
    effects of, 9, 11, 50, 71
air travel, dry air, 23
allergic rhinitis. *see* hay fever
allergies. *see also* asthma; hay fever
    and sinusitis, 32, 34
Aloe Vera Handbook (Skousen), 60
aloe vera juice, 60
antibiotics
    bacterial resistance, 38–40
    and sinusitis, 34
antihistamine medicine, 60
asthma
    and air pollution, 11, 71
    and sinusitis, 34
    treatment of, 41, 49, 61
Ayurveda medicine, 11, 60

B

Back to Eden (Kloss), 60
bacterial resistance, 38–40
blood
    circulation, 31, 41
    flow cycle, 18
brain
    direct nerve connections, 21
    infections, 31
breathing process, 18, 20, 65

C

cautery surgery, 38

tear ducts, 18, 56
traditional medicine
    Ayurveda, 11, 60
    Hatha Yoga, 11, 31, 65–66
    use of salt, 45
tuberculosis, 39
turbinates, 17, 19fig
    enlarged, 37–38, 59

V

ventilation, 37, 73

W

water, filtered, 51
water flow
    Stage I Jala Neti, 55
    Stage II Jala Neti, 55, 68
    problems, 58–59
Waterpik®, 54, 55
water temperature, 51

Y

yoga teaching
    breathing, 18, 20, 65
    Hatha Yoga, 11, 31, 65–66
    and Jala Neti, 9, 11, 51, 55, 68
    and Neti, 65–68
    seven paths, 31

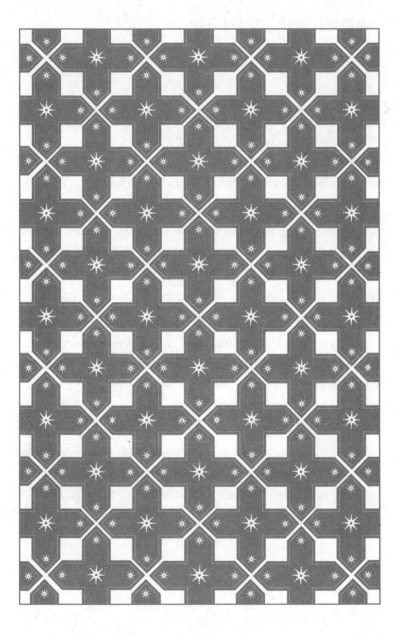

ABOUT THE AUTHOR

Warren Jefferson is a research writer, photographer, and graphic designer. As a long time partner in Book Publishing Company, he lends his photography and design skills to many books on health and diet, vegetarianism and green living, and Native American titles.

Warren's second book, *Colloidal Silver Today*, offers the latest findings and research on the low-tech alternative germ killer colloidal silver. It includes instructions for building a low-cost generator to produce colloidal silver at home for pennies an ounce.

Warren has been interested in Native American culture since first reading *Black Elk Speaks* in the '60s. His first book *The World of Chief Seattle*, is an historical account of Chief Seattle's people, the Suquamish, from pre-contact time to the present, and includes the only version of Chief Seattle's famous speech that is authorized by the Suquamish. The book was written in cooperation with the Suquamish tribe and they receive a portion of the royalties.

Warren and his wife Barbara have four children and are founding members of an intentional community in Tennessee, called The Farm, which is dedicated to promoting an awareness of ecology, vegetarianism, natural childbirth, and nonviolence. He is active in the local community and works with the local Victim Offender Reconciliation Program as a certified mediator helping people resolve conflicts and differences without going to court.

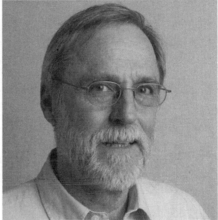

NOTES

BOOK PUBLISHING COMPANY

since 1974—books that educate, inspire, and empower

To find your favorite health books online, visit:
www.healthy-eating.com

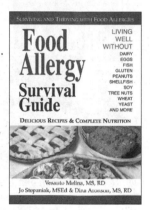

Food Allergy Survival Guide
Vesanto Melina, RD,
Jo Stepaniak, MSEd,
Dina Aronson, MS, RD
978-1-57067-163-0 $19.95 US

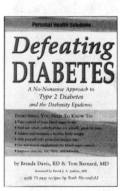

Defeating Diabetes
Brenda Davis, RD
Tom Barnard, MD
978-1-57067-139-5
$14.95 US

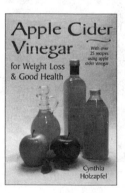

Apple Cider Vinegar for Weight Loss
& Good Health
Cynthia Holzapfel
978-1-57067-127-2 $9.95 US

Purchase these health titles from your local bookstore or
natural food store, or you can buy them directly from:

Book Publishing Company • P.O. Box 99 • Summertown, TN 38483
1-800-695-2241

Please include $3.95 per book for shipping and handling.

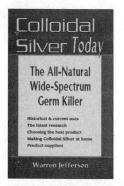
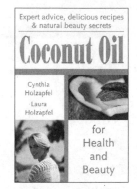
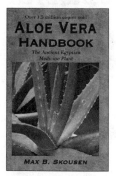
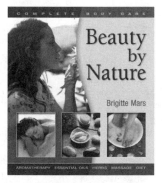